SUMMARY
Study Guide

BRAIN MAKER

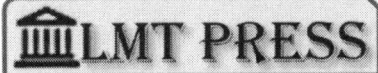

Copyright © 2015 by Lee Tang
Published by
LMT Press
Toronto, Canada
LMTPress.wordpress.com
LMTPress@gmail.com

Please note that this is an UNOFFICIAL summary study guide. This summary study guide is not affiliated, authorized, approved, licensed, or endorsed by the subject book's author or publisher. This book is NOT meant to be read as a replacement of the book which it summarizes but, instead, a supplement for review of the original book's main premises and to provide commentary and additional resources.

No part of this publication may be reproduced, stored in a retrieval system, or transmitted in any form or by any means, electronic, mechanical, photocopying, scanning, recording, or otherwise, except as permitted under Sections 107 or 108 of the 1976 United States Copyright Act, without either the prior written authorization from the publisher or author, except in the case of brief quotations permitted by copyright law.

First Edition: December, 2015
Issued in print and electronic formats.
ISBN 978-1-522-78130-1 (paperback)
ISBN 978-0-994-76404-1 (ebook)

Limit of Liability/Disclaimer of Warranty

The publisher and author make no representations or warranties with respect to the accuracy or completeness of these contents and disclaim all warranties such as warranties of fitness for a particular purpose. The author or publisher are not liable for any damages whatsoever. The fact that an individual or organization is referred to in this document as a citation or source of information does not imply that the author or publisher endorses the information that the individual or organization provided. The website addresses listed in the book were correct at the time going to print. However, the publisher and author are not responsible for the content of third-party websites, which are subject to change.

Your Free Gift

As a way of saying thanks for your purchase, I'm offering you a free book: How and When to Be Your Own Doctor by Isabelle Moser with Steve Solomon.

Isabelle Moser was born in 1940 and died in 1996. She had been fending off cancer since its first blow up when she was 26 years old. Coping with her own dicey health had been a major motivator for her interest in healing others. She will tell you more about it in this book.

The greatest accomplishment of her 56 years was to meld virtually all available knowledge about health and healing into a workable and most importantly, a simple model that allowed her to have amazing success. Her "system" is simple enough that even a generally well-educated non-medico can grasp it. And use it without consulting a doctor every time a symptom appears.

To claim your free gift, please subscribe to the newsletter by clicking here (http://bit.ly/1LpemFn).

Also by LMT Press

Dual Momentum Trend Trading: *How to Avoid Costly Trading Mistakes and Make More Money in the Stock, ETF, Futures and Forex Markets with This Simple and Reliable Swing Trading Strategy.*
http://amzn.to/1IZxbNI

Canada's Public Pension System Made Simple: *The Secrets To Maximizing Your Retirement Income From Government Pensions*
http://amzn.to/1Q9x2JR

Preface

Please note that this guide is a summary of the original book, "*Brain Maker: The Power of Gut Microbes to Heal and Protect Your Brain - for Life*", by Dr. David Perlmutter. It is a supplement to the original book, to make its main ideas easier to understand and put to practice.

About the Original Book

The rates of prevalence of chronic debilitating diseases such as autism, depression, Alzheimer's, and dementia are increasing. But advances in preventing and treating these diseases are almost nonexistent. The truth is, most doctors are trained to treat the *symptoms*, not the cause, of the *disease*; not seeking for ways to prevent it.

The good news is that a medical revolution is under way that will forever change how we understand, prevent, and treat these diseases. In his book, Dr. David Perlmutter explained in detail:

- The power of the new science by drawing on key clinical and laboratory studies and remarkable results from doctors and patients around the world,
- How lifestyle choices such as diet, exercise, sleep, and stress management influence our brain health and genetic expressions, and
- The essential keys to nourishing a healthy microbiome.

It is important to stay in charge of your healthcare through continued education and involvement. I recommend that you study Dr. Perlmutter's book and apply the ideas from the book to prevent and heal the debilitating illnesses that threaten you and your loved ones.

The purpose of this guide is to help you understand and practice the ideas described in the book. It includes:

- A **compact summary** of the original book. The summary will help you understand the key ideas and recommendations. It helps you master the concept while offering a rapid refresher when you need it most. Use it to keep the topic relevant and in front of you for times you fall off track. It'll save you precious time rereading the book to reabsorb, remember and recategorize. We did the work for you.

- **Online Materials**. These are extra learning materials such as on-demand replay of public lectures, and seminars on the topics covered in the chapter. They help reinforce your understanding of the ideas and make them easier to put to practice.

This guide is for you if you:

- Value time spent on EXECUTION, not reading
- Want to understand the key ideas of the book quickly
- Want a rapid refresher when needed

This study guide is more than a book summary: use it as a supplement to the book to make the ideas easier to understand and put to practice.

Table of Contents

YOUR FREE GIFT III

ALSO BY LMT PRESS IV

PREFACE V

INTRODUCTION 1

CHAPTER 1 YOUR MICROBIAL FRIENDS FROM BIRTH TO DEATH 3

CHAPTER 2 THE NEW SCIENCE OF INFLAMMATION 6

CHAPTER 3 WHY ANGRY GUTS MAKE FOR MOODY AND ANXIOUS MINDS 9

CHAPTER 4 HOW YOUR INTESTINAL FLORA CAN MAKE YOU FAT AND BRAINSICK 12

CHAPTER 5 AUTISM AND THE GUT 16

CHAPTER 6 THE TRUTH ABOUT FRUCTOSE AND GLUTEN 19

CHAPTER 7 COMMON EXPOSURES THAT MAKE A GOOD MICROBIOME GO BAD 22

CHAPTER 8 SIX ESSENTIAL KEYS TO BOOSTING YOUR BRAIN BY BOOSTING YOUR GUT 24

CHAPTER 9 THE GUIDE TO SUPPLEMENTS 27

CHAPTER 10 THE BRAIN MAKER 7-DAY MEAL PLAN 29

EPILOGUE 31

SUGGESTED REFERENCES 32

REVIEW REQUEST 33

INDEX 34

Introduction

Over the past century, scientists have made great progress in preventing and treating many life-threatening diseases such as smallpox, cholera, and scarlet fever. But they made little progress in preventing and treating debilitating diseases such as autism, attention deficit hyperactivity disorder (ADHD), dementia, multiple sclerosis, depression, Parkinson's, and Alzheimer's disease. Although doctors are prescribing drugs for patients with such diseases, the drugs don't work because many of these drugs don't treat the disease, just the symptoms. People who suffer from these diseases face several challenges that take an extensive toll on their health and finances. It is sad to see that, over the past twenty years, the prevalence of these diseases has reached epidemic levels, increasing the burden to the society.

Now the good news: new medical research has discovered the fundamental role of our microbiome in influencing health and longevity. In particular, scientists understand that an imbalance in the gut can cause brain disease, and restoring its balance may lead to cures. Over the past few years, we have seen many patients recovering from brain diseases by applying strict dietary disciplines to restore the health of their guts.

The human body comprises ten trillion cells, but harbors one hundred trillion invisible organisms or microbes, most are bacteria living in the gut. Scientists call this microbial community the microbiome. The gut microbiome performs many important functions to support our health and influence our gene expressions. It is so important to our health the National Institutes of Health launched the Human Microbiome Project in 2008 as an extension to the Human Genome Project.

The purpose of the book is to explain the new science, and recommend a practical program to help you prevent and treat these debilitating illnesses.

Online Materials

The gut flora: You and your 100 trillion friends (http://bit.ly/21w5pyA)

Human Microbiome Project (http://hmpdacc.org/)

Chapter 1
Your Microbial Friends from Birth to Death

The moment we enter the world, microbes colonize our bodies. Babies pick up microbes from their mothers and the environment. Studies show that early infant experiences, such as delivery by C-section, not being breast-fed, or exposures to antibiotics, can hurt the infant's microbiome. Disruption of the infant's microbiome can lead to inflammation and immune problems such as allergies, asthma, and even cancer later in life.

Why does the gut microbiome exert so much influence on our health? Because the good bacteria in the gut produce many important chemicals that help to curb inflammatory and immune responses - two central ingredients to prevent chronic illnesses. We need plenty of good bacteria in our gut to keep our brain healthy.

Important Roles Played by the Gut Flora:
- Digest and absorb nutrients from food.
- Neutralize toxins from the food that entered the gut.
- Support and influence the immune response.
- Protect the integrity of the intestinal wall so toxins cannot enter the bloodstream and invade the brain.
- Produce chemicals important for the health of the immune system, gut lining, and brain.
- Handle stress through their influence on the hormonal system.
- Control inflammation.
- Help you fall into sleep.

The gut has its own nervous system called "the second brain" by scientists. It can communicate with the brain and the central nervous system over the vast network of vagus nerves. Recent research shows the second brain can control many immune and hormonal functions without help from the main brain.

The gut is our first line of defense against toxic chemicals and germs because the gut-associated lymphatic tissue is a major part of the body's immune system. It attacks and defends against toxic chemicals found in the gut.

In a study published in 2013, scientists compared the rates of prevalence of Alzheimer's disease in people from 192 countries around the world. They found out that countries with the least sanitation had lower rates of Alzheimer's. And in countries with higher degrees of sanitation, people had less diversity of gut bacteria, and higher rates of Alzheimer's. This does not mean attention to hygiene causes Alzheimer's. It highlights that people growing up in countries with high degrees of sanitation have less diversity of gut bacteria to defense against disease. People in countries with lower degree of sanitation have more diversity of gut bacteria to defense against disease.

The Three Forces that Could Hurt Our Microbiome

1. Exposure to substances that disrupt the gut flora - they include environmental chemicals, ingredients in the food (e.g., sugar, gluten), water (e.g., chlorine), and drugs such as antibiotics.
2. Lack of nutrients for the beneficial gut bacteria
3. Stress.

Online Materials

The Invisible Universe Of The Human Microbiome (http://bit.ly/1NI68bH)

The human microbiome and what we do to it (http://bit.ly/1TlzGKD)

Chapter 2
The New Science of Inflammation

Inflammation is the immune system's response to injury or infection. It is the body's attempt to protect you and start the healing process. The normal signs of acute inflammation are: redness, swelling, heat, sometimes the loss of function, and mild to extreme pain. These symptoms will subside when that part of the body is healed.

When inflammation is out of control, it will cause a progressive destruction of normal tissues deep inside the body, causing serious illnesses. Sometimes there are no normal signs of inflammation such as pain or swelling, making it difficult to spot. But we can measure the chemicals that participate in the inflammation process and use them as markers. One such marker is the chemical TNF-α which plays an important role in inflammation throughout the body. With Alzheimer's disease, for example, the inflammation is taking place in the patient's brain. We can measure the TNF-α level in the brain and use it to predict cognitive decline and the risk of dementia.

Sugar is the culprit for most chronic illnesses. Excess sugar in the bloodstream can combine with proteins and fat to form compounds (AGEs) that could set off inflammation. It can also cause gut flora imbalance, triggering inflammation that could lead to type-2 diabetes and related complications. For people with genetic predispositions to these diseases, studies show they can support the good genes, while suppressing the bad, by keeping healthy blood sugar levels.

The Dangers of a Leaky Gut

A permeable or leaky gut allows various proteins in the gut to enter the bloodstream that leads to other parts of the body and the brain. This turns on an immune response that fuels a continuous state of inflammation, which can cause the blood-brain barrier to become permeable, resulting in leaky brains. A leaky brain is the cause for many neurological and autoimmune disorders.

LPS – the Responsible Villain

LPS (Lipopolysaccharide) is a part of the membrane of plenty of bacteria in the bowel. It protects the bacteria from being digested in the gut. Normally, the gut lining blocks the large LPS molecules from entering the bloodstream. But, if the gut lining is leaky or permeable, the LPS molecules can enter the bloodstream, increasing the LPS level in the bloodstream. In other words, high level of LPS in the blood is indicative of gut permeability.

Scientists are now using LPS to trigger inflammation in laboratories when they study the connection between gut permeability and chronic illnesses. In recent studies, they found out that:

Injection of LPS into the laboratory animals' body (not brain) can cause Alzheimer's disease.

Patients with ALS (Lou Gehrig's disease) have high levels of LPS in their blood, which correlate with the severity of the disease.

The Top Three Ways Your Gut Flora Can Reduce the Risk of Brain Disease

1. Inhibit inflammatory chemicals in the body.
2. Strengthen the integrity of the intestinal wall and prevent gut permeability.
3. Produce important chemicals for brain health, including BDNF, vitamin B12, and neurotransmitters such as glutamate and GABA.

Inflammation, the Gut, and the Mitochondria

Mitochondria are the tiny organisms found in the cells of the body, generating energy for the cells. Besides producing energy for the cells, they also play a big role in ridding the body of cancer cells. Unfortunately, mitochondria can easily be damaged by inflammation caused by an imbalanced microbiome. Dysfunctional mitochondria can destroy nerve cells, causing neurological disorders such as autism, multiple sclerosis, Alzheimer's, Parkinson's, and Lou Gehrig's disease. The good news is that we can make lifestyle changes to restock the mitochondria and strengthen this important part of the microbiome.

Online Materials

Mind-altering microbes: how the microbiome affects brain and behavior (http://bit.ly/1XzT0dy)

Leaky Gut Syndrome (http://bit.ly/1O4YIcM)

Minding your mitochondria (http://bit.ly/1IpQShp)

MS: The Basics - Symptoms of Multiple Sclerosis (http://bit.ly/1O4YPoK)

MS: The Basics – What Causes Multiple Sclerosis? (http://bit.ly/1RnZUO0)

Chapter 3
Why Angry Guts Make for Moody and Anxious Minds

Depression

Depression is an extended period of despair, hopelessness, and helplessness. The symptoms include distress, fatigue, loss of memory, anger, and unable to sleep. Today, mood and anxiety disorders are reaching epidemic levels. About one in four US adults suffers from mood disorders, and many are taking prescription drugs to treat the disease. But the drugs don't work because they don't treat the cause of the disease, just the symptoms, with serious side effects.

Depression is not a disorder caused by unbalanced brain chemicals, but an inflammatory disease caused by gut permeability. What causes gut permeability? Studies show it is our high-carb, low-fiber Western diet. High blood sugar is the biggest risk factor. A landmark study published in 2010 showed the increase in depression correlates with the increase in diabetes and obesity.

In a large study performed in 2013, the researchers found out that people with a history of autoimmune diseases and infections were more likely to develop mood disorders. This is because the medications and antibiotics that were used to treat the illnesses upset the balance of gut flora and caused mood disorders.

Change Your Gut, Change Your Mood

In 2011, researchers from McMaster University in Canada showed the gut can communicate with the brain and influence behavior. They used mice in the experiments and showed that they could alter the mice's behavior by changing their gut bacteria.

In 2013, a team of UCLA researchers showed that people who ate probiotics were more responsive to the cognitive region of the brain. And people who ate none were more responsive to the emotion-sensation region.

The gut-brain connection works both ways, creating a vicious cycle whereby stress and anxiety increase the stress hormone. And the increase in stress hormone leads to more inflammation and gut leakiness, which cause more stress and anxiety.

The Gut Bacteria and a Good Night's Sleep

The body produces a stress hormone cortisol in sync with our body clock, with levels lower at night and highest during the day. The gut bacteria, in concert with the levels of cortisol, stimulate production of chemicals important for inducing sleep. Disruption of the gut bacteria can have significant negative effects on sleep.

Anxiety

Anxiety disorders affect 40 million US adults. It's common to suffer from both anxiety and depression at the same time. The main difference between the two disorders is that anxiety is fear of the future, expecting something unfavorable; while depression doesn't entail such fears - just hopelessness.

Like depression, anxiety disorder is an inflammatory disease. People with anxiety disorder have:

Higher levels of inflammation and gut permeability,

Lower levels of BDNF,

Higher levels of stress hormone, and

An over-reactive stress response.

In a 2011 study, researchers showed that mice fed probiotics had lower levels of stress hormones, and behaved with less stress, anxiety and depression than mice fed plain food. In another study using human, researchers found that people who ate prebiotics (food for probiotics) displayed less stress and anxiety.

Children with ADHD

Today, more than 11 percent of kids aged 4 to 17 have ADHD, and two-third of them are taking drugs. ADHD and depression both have the same symptoms and the same underlying: unhealthy gut microbiome, chronic inflammation and leaky gut.

Researchers showed that many kids with ADHD were sensitive to gluten, dairy, and processed products with artificial ingredients and food colorings. That explains why ADHD kids have many bowel complaints such as chronic constipation, and loss of bowel control. When they put the kids with gluten-sensitivity on a gluten-free diet, the kids' behavior and functioning improved. This leads them to think that ADHD is not a separate disorder, but the symptoms of a disease caused by inflammation triggered by food sensitivity and an unhealthy gut microbiome.

Many ADHD kids don't have enough GABA, an important neurotransmitter, in their brain. This makes that area of the brain hyperactive, causing excessive movement characteristics of people with Tourette Syndrome. Researchers found out that they could fix the kids' GABA deficiency by feeding them with probiotics that could produce a lot of GABA.

Recent studies show that researchers can improve many kids' ADHD symptoms with dietary changes. So, instead of treating ADHD kids with dangerous drugs, we should treat them with dietary changes.

Online Materials

The Marketing of Madness: The Truth About Psychotropic Drugs (http://bit.ly/1SxWfLP)

David Perlmutter: Belly and the Brain (http://bit.ly/1YJ8WXW)

Depression, The Microbiome and Leaky Gut (http://bit.ly/1Q1DZfX)

How Gut Inflammation Triggers Depression (http://bit.ly/1PxrVDj)

How Gut Bacteria Affects Mood, Anxiety, and Weight (http://bit.ly/1QfQGm0)

The Gut-Brain Connection- ADHD & Autism can be healed today! (http://bit.ly/1Ro6MuI)

Chapter 4
How Your Intestinal Flora Can Make You Fat and Brainsick

Body mass index (BMI) (http://bit.ly/1HH5lFF) is a common measure of obesity. You are considered obese if your BMI is bigger than 30; overweight if between 25 and 30. Today, over 67 percent of US adults are overweight or obese, and 26 percent of US children are obese.

Overweight and obesity increase the risk of cardiovascular disease, cancer, diabetes, osteoarthritis, chronic kidney disease, and brain diseases. Obesity during pregnancy harms the developing fetus, putting the youngster at risk of obesity and diabetes later in life.

Obesity is an Inflammatory Disease

Fat tissues are bad because they produce pro-inflammatory chemicals, or cytokines, that increase the risk of dementia. Visceral fat, the excess fat around your belly, is dangerous because it dumps all the chemicals in the liver, causing inflammation and hormone-disruptions in the liver. In fact, a study published in 2005 showed that people with high waist-to-hip ratio (http://bit.ly/1QfQX8w) ratios had increased risk of shrinking brains, small strokes, and neurological disorders.

Blood Sugar and the Brain

Your blood sugar level rises after you ate carbohydrate foods. The rise in blood sugar triggers the body to produce insulin. Insulin regulates blood sugar by transporting excess glucose from the bloodstream into cells throughout the body where it will be used as fuel, or stored as fat.

When a cell is healthy, it has no problem responding to insulin. However, after a period of high insulin levels, the cells become insulin resistant. That means the cells will need more insulin to remove the excess glucose from the bloodstream. This sets in motion a vicious cycle whereby insulin resistance causes insulin level to increase, and the increased insulin level causes more insulin resistance. The cycle continues until your body cannot produce enough insulin to remove the excess glucose from the bloodstream, resulting in persistent high blood sugar levels. Eventually, this will progress to type 2 diabetes, a leading cause of early death, coronary heart disease, stroke, kidney disease, blindness and other neurological disorders.

Surges in blood sugar cause inflammation, which causes the depletion of important neurotransmitters and other minerals, harming both your nervous system and the liver. Excess sugar in the bloodstream can combine with proteins and fat to form compounds (AGEs) that could cause brain shrinkage. It also increases the insulin in your body, throwing the overall hormonal system off balance. As a so-called anabolic hormone, insulin encourages cell growth, promotes fat formation, and stimulates more inflammation. Even slight blood sugar issues below the threshold for diabetes can increase the risk for obesity, brain shrinkage, and Alzheimer's disease.

It is clear that high carbohydrate consumption contributes to diabetes. The diabetes (and obesity) epidemic started when the American Heart Association and the American Diabetes Association recommended the low-fat high-carb food pyramid to Americans three decades ago. Today, one out of eleven US adults has diabetes, and 28 percent of those people don't even know it.

Fat Tribes vs. Thin Tribes

There are thousands of species of gut bacteria, the two largest groups are: *Firmicutes* and *Bacteroidetes*. Firmicutes specialize in extracting calories (energy) from food and encourage fat storage. Studies show that high levels of Firmicutes have negative impacts on our metabolism and genetic expressions, which can lead to obesity, diabetes, cardiovascular disease, and inflammation. Bacteroidetes specialize in breaking down plant starches and fibers into shorter fatty acids the body can use as energy. The ratio between these two groups of bacteria (the F/B ratio) is an important obesity marker.

In a Harvard study published in 2010, the researchers compared the gut bacteria of children in rural Africa, where being obese or overweight is rare, to the European population. They found out that European microbiome lacked diversity and had more Firmicutes than Bacteroidetes. They also found out the Africans had more butyric and acetic acid and less propionic acid. High levels of propionic acid mean the gut has more harmful bacteria than friendly bacteria. These dissimilarities in the gut bacteria are due to diet differences. The African diet is high-fiber, low-sugar while the European is the opposite.

The study of twins published in 2013 showed similar results. When they transferred gut bacteria from an obese human twin into the guts of slender mice, the mice grew fat, and their gut flora became less diverse. But when they transferred gut bacteria from the thin twin to the lean mice, the mice stayed lean so long as they ate a healthy diet.

The Power of Diet

Recent studies show that an unhealthy diet can prevent good gut bacteria to do its work in keeping the body lean. In another study with mice using probiotics, the researchers found out that:

The mice that ate a "fast-food" diet – one high in unhealthy fat and sugar and low in fiber and vitamin B and D – grew obese.

The mice that got three servings per week of probiotic yogurt remained lean even though they were on the same fast-food diet.

The Power of Exercise

Recent studies involving professional athletes show that:

Exercise increases the diversity of the gut bacteria, and

Influences the gut's balance of bacteria to favor species that prevent weight gain.

Blame the Bugs, Not the Bonbon's

Microbiome plays a fundamental role in our body's energy dynamics, which affects the calories-in/calories-out equation. They influence the way we store fat, balance the glucose in our blood, and respond to the hormones that make us feel hungry or full. The diversity and composition of our gut bacteria are important. Studies show that higher F/B ratios correlate with higher risk for diabetes, obesity and gut permeability.

In 2014, a researcher from the University of Amsterdam showed that he could treat the blood sugar mayhem found in type 2 diabetes using fecal transplantation. He also used this procedure to improve insulin sensitivity. This ground breaking research may lead to effective ways of treating and preventing type 2 diabetes and related complications, including brain disorders.

Online Materials

What is Insulin Resistance and How to Avoid it (http://bit.ly/1IGfmOm)

How Our Gut Bacteria Control Body Weight (http://bit.ly/1IFioCw) – Interview with Dr. Gerard Mullin

Why We Get Fat and What To Do About It (http://bit.ly/1TxirGE) - A Conversation with Gary Taubes

The Complete Skinny on Obesity (http://bit.ly/1Nroxro)

Chapter 5
Autism and the Gut

Autism and autism spectrum disorder (ASD) are general terms used to describe a large and diverse family of complex brain disorders characterized by:

Difficulties in social interaction,

Challenges with verbal and nonverbal communications, and

Repetitive behaviors.

Today, about one out of 68 American children has the disorder, reflecting a tenfold increase over the past forty years.

Autism is not a single disease, and so no single cause. Studies have shown that autism isn't inherited, and environmental factors play a major role. Most kids with autism have an early life history of at least one or two traumas. These events not only influence a child's developing immune system and brain, they also affect the developing microbiome.

Gut Dysfunction Contributing to Brain Dysfunction

Multiple studies show that children with autism suffer from constipation, diarrhea, abdominal pain and bloating. Other research has determined that many individuals with autism have leaky guts. Due to these findings, experts now recommend a gluten-free diet for children with autism in order not to threaten their gut wall.

Research is finding the gut flora of individuals with autism differs from individuals without autism. In particular, people with autism have more clostridial species and less beneficial bacteria species. The most famous clostridial species of bacteria are the C. diff. These bacteria produce toxins, which can damage the bowel and cause diarrhea.

In a 2000 study published by Dr. Richard Sandler, he presented evidence that disruptions in gut flora may cause autism; and treating the disruption can ease the symptoms. In the study, he described the case of

Andy Bolte which became the highlight of the documentary called *The Autism Enigma*.

The PPA Link

Gut bacteria produce short-chain fatty acids as a by-product of fermentation of dietary fibers in the gut. Different gut bacteria produce different fatty acids. Butyric acid is the most beneficial fatty acid produced by gut bacteria. It helps to protect the integrity of the gut wall and is the primary energy source for the cells lining the colon. Clostridial species produce plenty of propionic acid (PPA), which, if allowed into the bloodstream, can cause mitochondrial dysfunction, leading to autism.

In studies done by a research group at the University of Western Ontario, researcher found that they could induce autism in mice by feeding them diets high in PPA. They could also induce autism by injecting PPA into the animals. They suggested the use of supplements such as NAC (n-acetyl cysteine) to counter the effects of PPA and reverse the damages.

Autism as a Mitochondrial Disorder

Autism is rare in countries such as Cambodia, a place with low sanitation than Western nations, because people living in places with low sanitation have more diversity of gut flora to defense against diseases.

In 2012, researchers at UC Davis discovered the connection between mitochondrial dysfunction and autism. They found out that many children with autism could not produce enough cellular energy, indicative of dysfunctional mitochondrial. This means that they don't have enough energy to power the brain, leading to autism. Environmental conditions can cause mitochondrial damage with varying degrees, resulting in a wide range of the autistic symptoms.

Taking Control of Your Genes

Although genes encoded by DNA are static, the expression of those genes is highly dynamic in response to environmental influences. Epigenetics is the study of sections of the DNA that activate or suppress the expression of particular genes. Environmental factors such as diet, nutrition, exercise, stress, sleep, and exposure to toxic chemicals all play a role in shaping the epigenome, which can change gene expression and cause brain disease. By taking control over all these factors, we can positively influence the epigenome and reduce the chances of getting brain disorder.

Online Materials

What is Autism? Do you know the signs? (http://bit.ly/1PxE778)

Autism - what we know (and what we don't know yet) (http://bit.ly/1MXmoSV)

Autism - The Fundamental Role of Gut Bacteria (http://bit.ly/1O5gih2)

Autism Enigma (available only in Canada) (http://bit.ly/1TxkOEz)

Mitochondrial Dysfunction in Autism Spectrum Disorders (http://bit.ly/1jBos8u)

The Epigenome at a Glance (http://bit.ly/1jAU4Lp)

Insights From Identical Twins (http://bit.ly/1jAG6cm)

Chapter 6
The Truth about Fructose and Gluten

Fructose

Studies show that eating too much fructose can lead to serious health problems such as high blood sugar, high blood fats, and high blood pressure. High fructose levels can cause gut bacteria to pass through the intestinal wall into the bloodstream, and damage the liver.

Here are three reasons fructose is bad:

High doses of fructose are a big burden to the liver which metabolizes the fructose. This exhausts the liver, and produces a toxic by-product uric acid, which causes high blood pressure, gout, and kidney stones.

Unlike glucose, fructose has no immediate impact on blood sugar levels, and so no impact on insulin and leptin. So you don't fill full and keep on eating. That's why diets high in fructose often lead to obesity and other metabolic disorders.

When the gut bacteria digest fructose, they release a mixture of gases, which can cause bloating, discomfort, or stomach pain.

Most of the fructose we consume today are from high-fructose corn syrup (HFCS), a sweetener found in sugar-sweetened drinks and processed foods. HFCS and table sugar have similar molecular structures - a mixture of about half fructose and half glucose. This makes HFCS and table sugar much worse than pure fructose because of the compound adverse effects of both glucose and fructose. The glucose part of the molecule spikes blood-sugar levels, which creates insulin resistance and exhausts the pancreas. The fructose part disrupts liver metabolism and produces toxic byproducts such as uric acid.

Natural whole fruits and vegetables are OK because they have relatively little fructose (or sugar) when compared with, say, a can of regular soda or concentrated juice. And the fiber in fruits and vegetables slows down absorption of fructose into the bloodstream.

Is artificial sweetener a safe and healthier alternative to real sugar? According to a 2013 study, people who drank artificially sweetened drinks had doubled the risk of developing diabetes than those who consumed sugar-sweetened drinks.

Gluten

Gluten is the protein found in wheat, barley, and rye. It comprises two main groups of proteins: glutenins and gliadins. Gluten is dangerous because its "sticky" nature interferes with the breakdown and absorption of nutrients, which leads to poor digestion. The body does not regard the poorly digested food as normal, so it sets off an alarm to the immune system. Once the alarm has sounded, the immune system sends out inflammatory chemicals that can damage tissues, leaving the walls of the intestine compromised, resulting in a leaky gut. Once you have a leaky gut, the LPS molecules in your gut can enter the bloodstream and travel to the brain. This can break down the blood-brain barrier, putting you at risk for cancer, brain, and autoimmune disease.

Gluten can cause celiac disease if it damages the absorptive surface of the small intestine so the body cannot absorb nutrient from food. Recent studies show that celiac disease contributes to an imbalance in the microbiome, which can intensify the disorder, creating a vicious cycle. Children delivered by C-section and those who've taken many antibiotics have a higher risk for the disease.

While only a small percentage of the population suffers from celiac disease, it's possible for everyone to have some degree of gluten sensitivity. Those who experience symptoms of gluten sensitivity complain of bowel trouble, such as stomach pain, nausea, diarrhea, and constipation. But those without the symptoms could experience a silent attack elsewhere in their body. That is why people call gluten a "silent germ" because it can inflict permanent damage without your knowing it.

A 2013 study shows that gluten can cause the onset of type 1 diabetes by changing the gut microbiome. A more recent study shows that gluten promotes weight gain and can contribute to type 2 diabetes.

Beware of gluten-free products. Many are made with refined, gluten-free grains low in fiber, vitamins, and other nutrients. They can be just as junky and nutrient-poor as processed products that don't come with a "gluten-free" label. It's better to eat real natural foods that are "gluten-free" than to eat processed foods that are labeled "gluten-free".

Online Materials

Fat Chance: Fructose 2.0 (http://bit.ly/1NqeiiK)

Dark Secrets of Artificial Sweeteners Revealed with Mike Adams (http://bit.ly/1Rohb9J)

Grain Brain: How Gluten Affects Your Brain & Beyond with Dr. David Perlmutter (http://bit.ly/1QVoerh)

Why Is Gluten So Bad? The Science Behind Gluten Intolerance (http://bit.ly/1XLe6QT)

How do you know if a food contains gluten? (http://bit.ly/1PxFhzv)

Gluten Free Diet Scam: Gluten Free Bread May Destroy Your Core Health! (http://bit.ly/1TCfggX)

Why Your Uric Acid Levels Matter (http://bit.ly/1N4C2cO)

Chapter 7
Common Exposures That Make a Good Microbiome Go Bad

Antibiotics

Antibiotics improve our lives by treating and preventing disease. They are also used in farming and agriculture to treat infections and improve yields. But widespread use of antibiotics has led to the increase in harmful antibiotic-resistant varieties that current antibiotics cannot touch. Recent studies show that use of antibiotics can increase the risk of breast cancer. Even short pulses of antibiotics can upset the balance of the gut microbiome, leading to brain diseases such as ADHD, and autism. So, we should avoid taking antibiotics and eat antibiotics-free meat.

The Pill

Birth control pills are synthetic hormones that have immediate biological effects on the human body. They will take a toll on the microbial community. Long-term use (more than 5 years) can cause:

Decreased thyroid hormone and testosterone in circulation

Increase insulin resistance, oxidative stress, and markers of inflammation

Depletion of certain vitamins, minerals, and antioxidants.

The most common side effects of using the Pill are mood and anxiety disorders; and recent studies show that using the Pills can increase the risk of Crohn's disease.

NSAIDS

Studies show that using nonsteroidal anti-inflammatory medications (NSAIDS), such as Advil and Aleve, can increase the risk of damage to the gut lining, especially when gluten is present.

Environmental Chemicals

Environmental chemicals are harmful because they accumulate in hormone glands and fat tissues. We are exposed to large amounts of toxic substances. For example, municipal water is over-treated with chemicals toxic to the gut bacteria. Certain fish have concentration of chemicals in their tissues. Many livestock eats grains sprayed with pesticides and herbicides, which accumulate in their body. Eating fish, meat and dairy can expose us to chemicals used along the food chain.

Herbicide-Laden GMO Foods

GMOs are plants or animals that have been genetically engineered with new genes from other organisms. Eighty percent of conventional processed food use GMOs. The two top GMO crops in the US are corn and soybean.

Using herbicide resistant GMO seeds has allowed farmers to use vast amounts of herbicides such as glyphosate. Studies showed a high correlation between the rates of prevalence of celiac disease and glyphosate applied to wheat. In a study published in 2013, researcher described how residual glyphosate changed the balance of gut bacteria, contributing to the increase in prevalence of gluten sensitivity.

Online Materials

Antibiotics in Agriculture: Are they making us fat? (http://bit.ly/1HHaltW)

Antibiotics fueling modern plagues (http://bit.ly/1O6OI2X)

The Problems with The Birth Control Pill (http://bit.ly/1Sy3DXJ)

Side-Effects of NSAIDs (http://bit.ly/1Q1KWhe)

The Health Dangers of Roundup (glyphosate) Herbicide (http://bit.ly/1NIyLpo)

Monsanto Documentary - This is a shocking video about the company (http://bit.ly/1MXnluu)

Chapter 8
Six Essential Keys to Boosting Your Brain by Boosting Your Gut

Key #1: Choose Foods Rich in Probiotics

Probiotic foods are rich in beneficial bacteria. Fermented foods are the best probiotic foods. It is the lactic acid fermentation that makes the food probiotic. In this process, good bacteria convert the sugar in the food into lactic acid. In doing so, the beneficial bacteria multiply and grow; and the lactic acid protects the fermented food from harmful bacteria.

Key #2: Go Low-Carb, Embrace High-Quality Fat

Ideal meal: Fill two-third of your plate with veggies, and the rest with roughly 3 to 4 ounces of protein.

Eat non-starchy veggies, low-sugar fruits, fermented foods, and healthy fats. Don't worry about the so-called "high-cholesterol" foods.

Use butter, extra-virgin olive oil, or coconut oil for cooking. Avoid processed oils such as vegetable oils.

Limit starchy vegetables, legumes, cow's milk and cream, non-gluten grains, natural sweeteners, chocolates, and whole sweet fruits.

Choose organic and non-GMO wherever possible.

Avoid Gluten. Choose foods that are naturally gluten-free, not products whose gluten has been processed out of the food.

Meat - choose antibiotic-free, grass-fed, 100 percent organic meats.

Fish - choose wild fish, which often have lower levels of toxins than farmed fish.

Key #3: Enjoy Wine, Tea, Coffee, and Chocolate

You can enjoy wine, coffee, and chocolate in moderation, and tea with no fear. They all contain polyphenols, which are powerful antioxidant found in plants. They play a role in preventing degenerative diseases such as cancer and cardiovascular diseases.

Key #4: Choose Foods Rich in Prebiotic

Prebiotics are foods for the helpful gut bacteria. They have three characteristics:

Non-digestible so they could pass through the stomach into the intestines without being digested.

Can be fermented or metabolized by the intestinal bacteria.

Offer health benefits to the body.

Recommend aiming for 12 grams daily, either from supplements or soluble fiber found in fruits and vegetables, or both.

Prebiotics help the friendly gut bacteria thrive, promote a healthier microbiome in the intestinal tract, and crowd out the harmful bacteria.

Key #5: Drink Filtered Water

To avoid environmental chemicals entering your food chain, consider:

Filter your water before you drink.

Opt for foods produced with the least amount of pesticides and herbicides.

Limit consumption of canned, processed, and prepared foods.

Never microwave foods in plastic containers.

Avoid storing foods in plastic containers and plastic wrap made from PVC (with recycling code "3").

Avoid plastic water bottles marked with a "PC" for polycarbonate, or the recycling label "7". Buy reusable bottles made of food-grade stainless steel or glass.

Don't use non stick / Teflon-coated pans or cooking utensil.

Key #6: Fast Every Season

Studies show that calorie restriction provides many health benefits. Intermittent fasting - stop eating for a day or two regularly - provides comparable health benefits and is a more practical strategy.

Recommend you fast at least four times a year: No food, but lots of water for a 24-hour period four times a year. If you take medications, continue to take them during the fasting period. If you take diabetes medications, you need to consult with your doctor first because you may need to adjust your medications when you fast.

Online Materials

What is Probiotic (http://bit.ly/1YJkKJE)

Top 10 PROBIOTICS Foods (http://bit.ly/1NIzGWW)

Prebiotics: What are they and why are they so important? (http://bit.ly/1Tmc748)

The many benefits of prebiotics (http://bit.ly/1OyNsu2)

Is Coffee Bad for You? (http://bit.ly/1Q1LB2j)

Why fasting bolsters brain power (http://bit.ly/1Rojeun)

Chapter 9
The Guide to Supplements

Probiotics: Five Core Species

Probiotics are live, friendly bacteria that live in the gut. There are thousands of different species of bacteria that make up the human microbiome, different strains offer different benefits. Most probiotic supplements contain several strains. Look for supplements that are marked *hypoallergenic* and contain at least the following species:

Lactobacillus plantarum: found in fermented vegetables.

Lactobacillus acidophilius: found in fermented dairy products.

Lactobacillus brevis: found in sauerkraut and pickles.

Bifidobacterium lactis (also called B. Animalis): found in fermented milk products.

Bifidbacterium longum

Other Supplements to Consider

DHA: Docosahexaenoic acid (DHA) is an omega-3 fatty acid that makes up more than 90 percent of the omega-3 fats in the brain. The richest source of DHA in nature is human breast milk. Take 1,000 mg daily.

Turmeric: Turmeric is a member of the ginger family and is the seasoning that gives curry powder the yellow color. If you're not eating a lot of curry dishes, take 500 mg twice daily.

Coconut oil: Take 1 or 2 teaspoons daily, or employ it when you cook food.

Alpha-lipoic acid: Take 300 mg daily.

Vitamin D: The body produces Vitamin D in the skin upon exposure to ultraviolet radiation from the sun. Take 5,000 IU daily.

Online Materials

Tourette's Syndrome - Life With Tourette's (http://bit.ly/1Sy4EPi)

3 things you need to know when choosing a probiotic supplement (http://bit.ly/1XIBr5R)

No Fear Enemas- For SUPER Gut Health (http://bit.ly/1lYBcYE)

Chapter 10
The Brain Maker 7-Day Meal Plan

Daily Menu Planning

When planning for your daily menu, follow the dietary guidelines outlined in chapter 8:

Eat at least one fermented food (probiotics), and 12 grams of prebiotics.

Fill two-third of your plate with veggies, and the rest with roughly 3 to 4 ounces of protein.

Use butter, extra-virgin olive oil, or coconut oil for cooking. Avoid processed oils such as vegetable oils.

Avoid processed foods, sugary drinks, sugar, flour, gluten, and starchy vegetables.

Drink only filtered water.

The 7-day Plan

This plan provides you with 7 days of concrete meal ideas. You can follow the plan if you sense the need to reboot your microbiome. When following this 7-day plan, don't be afraid to make replacements.

Before you start...

Buy your supplements and probiotics.

Fast for the 24 hours before day one.

Try a probiotic enema in the morning of day one.

During the week...

Perform aerobic exercise or brisk walking for at least 30 minutes every day.

Try to sleep and get up at the same time every day.

After the week...

Plan your daily menu following the dietary guidelines.

Repeat the 7-day meal plan when you sense the need to reboot your microbiome.

Online Materials

How to make Kefir at home, forever (http://bit.ly/1PxIAGX)!

How to Make Yogurt - Super Easy!!! (http://bit.ly/1N4DzQe)

Homemade Quark cheese (http://bit.ly/1MXoAcY)

How to Make Sauerkraut at Home (http://bit.ly/1QVrMcQ)

How to Make Kimchi (http://bit.ly/1Nqi5MZ)

How to Make Kombucha Tea (http://bit.ly/1OHmdf4)

Epilogue

Fecal Microbial Transplantation (FMT) is the latest advance in the battle against chronic illnesses. It involves the transfer of fecal matter from a carefully screened, healthy stool donor into the colon of a sick patient. It provides an opportunity to restore the health of the patient's microbiome, setting the stage for a return to a better health.

The procedure has shown remarkable results in treating a wide range of health conditions, including C. diff infection, Crohn's disease, celiac disease, multiple sclerosis and Tourette Syndrome. It has huge potential for managing and treating Alzheimer's, autism, diabetes, obesity, and Parkinson's disease.

Another therapy in development today is the use of parasitic worm eggs to cure inflammatory bowel disease (IBD). A small human trial shows that giving people the microscopic pig-whipworm eggs can reduce IBD symptoms. Exposures to these eggs helps to restore balance to the gut microbiome. Experiments are underway to see if the procedure applies to other diseases.

Online Materials

Dr. David Perlmutter's Brain Maker (http://bit.ly/1NrrGaG)

How Fecal Transplants Can Save Lives (http://bit.ly/1Iq5nBM)

Dr. Perlmutter: Brain Maker, Fecal Transplants, and How to Heal Your Gut with Real Food (http://bit.ly/1OHmuyn)

Suggested References

As I mentioned earlier in the guide, it is very important to stay in charge of your healthcare through continued education and involvement. I have listed below recent conferences on health subjects that might be of interest to you. I recommend you register for each of them. Registration is FREE and you will receive free replays from the conference.

Recommended Conferences

The Diabetes Bundle (http://bit.ly/1LXB9RC)

2015 Health Gut Summit (http://bit.ly/1XUAwPH)

2015 Diabetes Summit (http://bit.ly/1NDWfFG)

2015 Mental Wellness Summit (http://bit.ly/1NcMpeP)

2016 Heal Your Gut Summit (http://bit.ly/1OOZ2zw)

2016 Fat Summit (http://bit.ly/1OtCXJZ)

Recommended Reference for Gluten-Free Cooking

Gluten Free Teacher: Unlock the secrets of a Gluten Free Diet (http://bit.ly/1NgGgAA)

Felicity's Gluten Free Diet Handbook (http://bit.ly/1QBlw8V)

Gluten Demystified (http://bit.ly/1N5oxvS)

Gluten Free Cooking For A Healthier YOU! (http://bit.ly/1OcychR)

Gluten Free Cooking for Weight Loss (http://bit.ly/1Q9qfA3)

Gluten Free Creations, All Spiced Up! Certification (http://bit.ly/1IyulPv)

Gluten Free Life In Simple Steps (http://bit.ly/1NcEK06)

How to Navigate a Gluten Free Lifestyle (http://bit.ly/1TQeu05)

How to Quit Gluten & Become a Whole Foods Baking Expert (http://bit.ly/1PNPhEW)!

Online Pastry School - Gluten Free Bread Baking Course (http://bit.ly/1PNNOhL)

Review Request

Thank you for putting this study guide to work! I hope that the information is useful to you.

Before you go, I want you to do one thing- don't worry, it will only take about 2 minutes of your time, and it will help you.

I'd be grateful if you post an honest review of this book on Amazon, whether you loved or hated this book. I read all the reviews and this will allow me to pinpoint what you liked and disliked. Your review will help me see what is and isn't working so I can better serve you and all my other readers even more. By leaving a review you are helping yourself as it will allow me to get your feedback and make improvements in the next edition of the book.

Your support matters and it makes a difference.

If you'd like to leave a review then all you need to do is go to the review section of this book (http://amzn.to/1QFeyBb).

Thanks again for your support.

Index

acetic acid 13
ADHD 9
AGEs 5, 12
Alpha-lipoic acid 26
Alzheimer's disease 4
American Diabetes Association 12
American Heart Association 12
antibiotics 3
Antibiotics 21
Anxiety 9
artificial sweetener 19
ASD 15
Autism 15
autism spectrum disorder 15
Bacteroidetes 12
BDNF 9
Bifidbacterium longum 26
Bifidobacterium lactis 26
Birth control pills 21
Blood Sugar 11
Body mass index 11
breast-fed 3
butyric acid 13
C. diff 15
calories-in/calories-out equation 14
celiac disease 19
Clostridial species 16

Coconut oil 26
C-section 3
cytokines 11
Depression 8
DHA 26
diversity of gut bacteria 4
Environmental Chemicals 21
Epigenetics 17
epigenome 17
F/B ratio 13
fasting 25
fecal transplantation 14
Fecal Transplantation 30
Fermented foods 23
Firmicutes 12
FMT 30
food pyramid 12
Fructose 18
GABA 10
gliadins 19
gluten 9
Gluten 19
gluten sensitivity 19
gluten-free 10
gluten-free products 20
glutenins 19
gluten-sensitivity 10
glyphosate 22
GMO 22

Gut Flora 3	permeable gut 5
Herbicide 22	power of Diet 13
HFCS 18	Power of Exercise 13
high-fructose corn syrup 18	PPA 16
Human Microbiome Project 1	Prebiotic 24
IBD 30	probiotic enema 28
Inflammation 5	probiotics 9, 10
inflammatory bowel disease 30	Probiotics 23
insulin 11	propionic acid 13
insulin resistant 11	sanitation 4
Intermittent fasting 24	second brain 3
Lactobacillus acidophilius 26	study of twins 13
Lactobacillus brevis 26	sugar 18
Lactobacillus plantarum 26	Sugar 5
leaky brain 5	sweetener 18
Leaky Gut 5	The 7-day Mean Plan 28
LPS 6	The Autism Enigma 16
microbiome 1	TNF-α 5
Mitochondria 6	Tourette Syndrome 10
Mitochondrial Disorder 16	Turmeric 26
NSAIDS 21	Visceral fat 11
Obesity 11	Vitamin D 26
Overweight 11	waist-to-hip ratio 11
parasitic worm eggs 30	

Made in the USA
San Bernardino, CA
29 April 2016